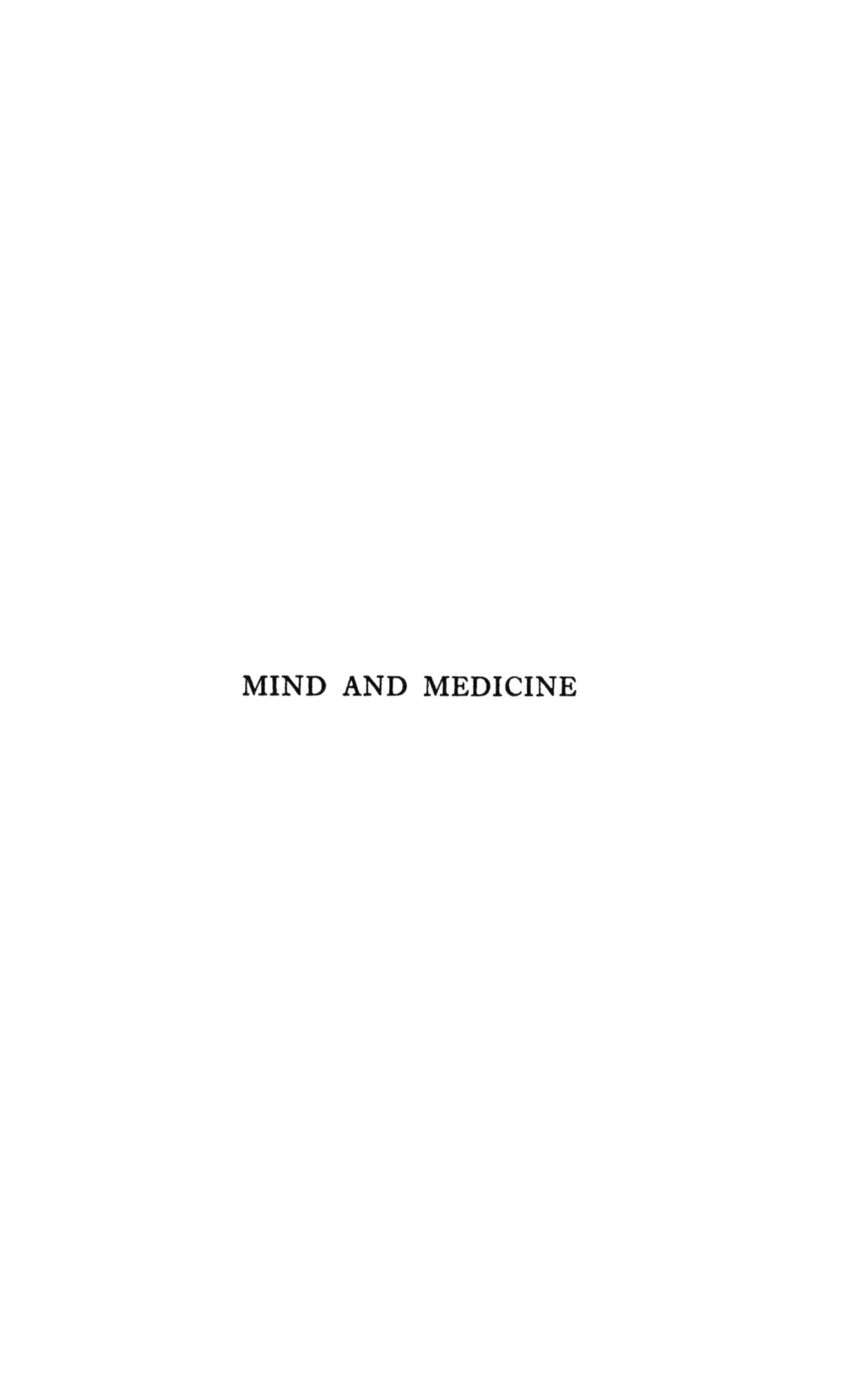

MIND AND MEDICINE

COLUMBIA UNIVERSITY PRESS
Columbia University
New York

SALES AGENTS
London
HUMPHREY MILFORD
Amen Corner, E.C.

Shanghai
EDWARD EVANS & SONS, Ltd.
30 North Szechuen Road

Mind and Medicine

By

THOMAS W. SALMON, M.D.

Professor of Psychiatry in Columbia University

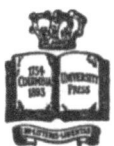

New York

COLUMBIA UNIVERSITY PRESS

1924

CONTENTS

Introduction...................... 1

Attitude of medicine toward insanity... 4

Attitude of medicine toward psychoneuroses....................... 7

Attitude of medicine toward other mental
problems...................... 13

Origin of present attitude of medicine
toward mind................... 14

Waning interest in function........... 17

Some new tendencies............... 22

Conclusion...................... 28

MIND AND MEDICINE*

It is customary to encourage the member of the faculty who has the honor of giving this address to look up from the bed or laboratory bench beside which he works and tell his fellow-craftsmen how the structure of scientific medicine growing under our hands appears from his particular point of view. In this he is like the workman on a great building who occasionally straightens his back and refreshes himself from toil by visualizing that which he is helping to build, in all its completed beauty, strength and usefulness. Here the simile fails, however, for it will not be given to those who to-day are building the structure of scientific medicine ever to see it completed. Neither can we, when our imagery is inadequate, stimulate it, like the mechanic, by a glimpse of the architect's

* Address at the opening session of the College of Physicians and Surgeons, Columbia University, September 26, 1923.

drawings, for we are helping to construct a living thing that changes as it grows and no architect has drawn its plans or prepared its specifications. Yet, changing as is the form of modern medicine and undetermined as are its ultimate dimensions, the spirit with which it is endowed and the purpose that motivates those who work upon it are unchanging. That spirit is the spirit of scientific investigation and that purpose is service to humanity. No material proffered by a fellow-workman can be rejected without careful examination if produced by scientific investigation and utilizable to promote the welfare of mankind. Every one of our fellow-workmen is entitled to point out what he conceives to be elements of strength or weakness in the structure to which he is devoting the best efforts of his life.

Recently, President Vincent traced, in a few clear and forceful paragraphs, the growth of medicine through its theological and metaphysical stages into its scientific stage.[1] He

[1] Vincent, George E., "The Rockefeller Foundation: a review for 1922," New York, 1923.

reminded us that to-day the practitioner, although thoroughly imbued with scientific spirit and familiar, through first-hand knowledge, with the scientific methods by which the information that he uses in his daily work has been acquired, nevertheless, still *practices an art*. He must add his own personal experiences and his own independent observations to the accumulated knowledge of anatomy, physiology, pharmacology, biochemistry, pathology and bacteriology to which he has fallen heir. In the end, not only the amount of practical service that scientific medicine can render but the extent of the public support that medical institutions will receive, depend upon the wisdom, skill and breadth of view with which the individual practitioner practices his art.

In this brief summary of medical progress, Dr. Vincent went on to say:

"It has been asserted with some reason that, in its preoccupation with the diseases of the body, scientific medicine has too much neglected the psychic and social factors. The rapid spread of cults which invoke various forms of mental suggestion, is probably due in some measure to the failure of modern medicine to include in its scope the relations of mental and physical states, to study these in a scientific spirit, and to utilize the healing powers of rationally controlled suggestion. Recent progress in psychiatry, the war-time experiences with disorders of the mind, the rise of mental hygiene, and the increased attention being given these subjects in medical schools and at professional meetings are evidences that the mental aspect of disease is being recognized more fully."

It is possible to present at this time only a few of the numerous evidences supporting the opinion voiced by Dr. Vincent that scientific medicine has too much neglected the psychic factors in disease.

ATTITUDE OF MEDICINE TOWARD INSANITY

One of the saddest results of the failure of medical science and art to include mind in their interests is the amazingly small share of medical attention that is given to those grave and widely prevalent disorders to which the collective term "insanity" is applied. Few physicians are aware that one person in ten in this state who reaches adult life is admitted to a mental hospital before he dies or that the number of beds in public hospitals for the insane in this country equals those occupied by all other sick persons combined. This vast amount of illness is cared for by only a handful of medical workers, compared with the staffs of general hospitals, and even the names and chief characteristics of its most common forms are less well known to many well-educated physicians than are those of rare tropical diseases. The forty thousand patients with mental diseases in the public hospitals of this state present some exceedingly important problems for medical research, not only in the field of mental medicine but in that of general medical science, yet only a few thousand dollars are expended annually upon such research. Public opinion and the law recognize mental disease as a medical problem and almost invariably the physician is first appealed to when it appears in a family, but he is usually not only quick to admit his lack of information regarding the questions of prognosis and treatment about which the distressed family of the patient are anxiously inquiring but will often acknowledge to a colleague his profound lack of interest in everything that pertains to them. Physicians sign hundreds of certificates committing patients to mental hospitals to which they never even pay a casual visit, although they may be situated within the same city.

If the frank mental diseases constituted a special medical problem, having scarcely any points of contact with those occupying the attention of general medicine, it would be of little moment to anyone (except the unfortunate patients themselves) that the insane poor should be, for the most part, marooned on islands of their own, with those few physicians who elect to care for them. It happens, however, that some intensely interesting general medical problems are interwoven with the special ones of mental illness. The insane, whose mind processes are made accessible and "segregated," so to speak, by disease provide opportunities for the study, under exceedingly favorable conditions, of those relations between mental and physical states which Dr. Vincent reminds us have been overlooked in the growth of scientific medicine.

ATTITUDE OF MEDICINE TOWARD PSYCHO-NEUROSES

Although it has been possible virtually to exclude the mental disorders which we call "insanity" from the general interests of medicine, some other procedure was required in dealing with the states called psychoneuroses by physicians and "nervousness" by the public. Hysteria, neurasthenia, states of pathological anxiety, fear or doubt and morbid fixation of attention upon organs and functions of the body are far too widespread and their possessors make far too insistent demands upon the general medical profession to permit them to be ignored as insanity has been. The public chooses not to regard these disorders as "mental" and in this is aided by a medical reluctance to acknowledge them as such. No one can estimate their incidence. Dr. William J. Mayo said not long ago, "Neurasthenia, psychasthenia, hysteria and allied neuroses are the causes of more human misery than tuberculosis or cancer." We know that during the Great War, under the misleading designation of "shell shock" or the better one of "war neuroses," they constituted a drain upon man-power comparable only to that from wounds and the effects of gas. More than 200,000 men were discharged from active service, with these disorders, in the British Army alone.[2] They cloud the happy days of childhood, destroy the unity of families, dull the achievements of brilliant minds and replace the calm and serenity of old age with anxiety and fear.

It is easy to see why scientific medicine finds itself confronted by a dilemma in having

[2] Collie, Colonel Sir John, "Management of war neuroses and allied disorders in the army." Reprint 26 from *Mental Hygiene*, 2:1 –18, January, 1918.

to deal with such a great mass of mental illness as that constituted by the psycho-neuroses and at the same time to preserve its aloofness toward all problems in mind in relation to disease. Several compromises have resulted. By one of these compromises the disorder is forcibly transformed into one of the fairly well-understood forms of physical disease, and the mental symptoms considered as incidental and relegated to the background. Just what form of physical disease the psycho-neurosis is transformed into depends upon the direction of medical interest at the time. Uterine displacements, impacted molars and endocrine disorders have all served their turn. In this transformation, the patients' anxiety regarding their general health and the frequency with which their compulsive thinking fixes their attention upon the functioning of their organs help very materially. The physician is enabled to ignore the fact that the bodily symptoms so dramatically presented are mostly symbolic and is at liberty to treat them as if they were real. A colleague told me once that he curretted an old lady who had the delusion that she was pregnant, hoping thus to rid her mind of something she thought was in her uterus. This is an extreme example, perhaps, but the most amazing situations develop every day as the result of the general medical acceptance of physical life as the most convenient field of battle in dealing with the psychoneuroses. Two factors bid fair soon to dispose of this compromise, without the necessity of any deeper medical interest in mind than exists at present. One is the fact that hosts of quacks are prepared to conduct proceedings at this level much more successfully than the physicians. These competitors of ours are not greatly troubled by qualms of conscience, for forcing facts to meet situations is their daily task. Besides, they have not the underlying impatience with the psychoneurotic and his difficulties that handicaps the physician and, despite his efforts to conceal it, frequently interferes with professional relations. Remunerative patients with functional disorders are just as welcome to the quack as those with organic ones—perhaps more so. The other factor that must effectually modify the prevailing medical attitude toward the psychoneurotic and his woes is the element of time. The increasing shortage of physicians and increasing pressure upon scientifically trained practitioners will some day convince the profession generally of the tremendous economic waste involved in permitting itself to become a subsidized audience for the great dramatization of disease that the psychoneuroses constitute.

Another compromise in the medical dilemma created by such unorthodox diseases as the psychoneuroses is to refuse to accept the seductive invitations of psychoneurotic patients to deal with their disorders on the physiological level on which they best maintain themselves. This is often done by flatly denying the faithfulness of the picture presented—no matter how realistically it is

2

painted—and denouncing the patient (to himself and his family if not to the world at large)
as a simulator, who but for courtesy might be
stigmatized by a harsher word. This course
has several apparent advantages. It recog-
nizes the element of simulation even if it
places the blame where it does not belong.
It fills the denouncer with that thrill of self-
approval that comes to all of us when we
detect wrong-doing (of a sort that we do not
habitually commit) and can confront the cul-
prit with evidence of his misconduct. Its
effects upon patients, however, are apt to be
unfortunate. The human being who is ob-
sessed by a morbid anxiety that dogs his days
and nights and not infrequently makes death
preferable to life is bewildered when suddenly
accused of having conceived the thing deliber-
ately and continued it with a more or less
fraudulent intent. The hypochondriacal patient whose attention is so firmly attached to
his bodily functions that he can no longer
detach it and contemplate the beautiful things

in life which used to be the sources of his happiness is amazed to learn that he has not only accomplished the fixation himself (which may, indeed, be the case) but that he has done it knowingly and for a purpose that will not bear too close examination. Both these compromises are poor affairs, and their sadness is not lessened when we reflect that they are deemed necessary and ethically justifiable only because of an unfortunate point of view toward mind that grew up during the most brilliant and productive period of medical progress.

ATTITUDE OF MEDICINE TOWARD OTHER MENTAL PROBLEMS

It would not be without interest to trace some other results of that point of view. Important factors in the practical management of crime and delinquency have, with new knowledge in psychiatry, been found to lie within the field of medicine. New light upon the emotions has provided opportunities for physicians to render services to the family that may go far toward reestablishing the old and honorable position of the doctor as "guide, philosopher and friend." Over all these new opportunities for usefulness to men, women and children borne down by the stresses of life there hangs, however, the shadow that has been indicated in what I have said regarding the fundamental difference in the attitude of medicine toward data regarding bodily states and toward those relating to mental states. Let us devote no more time to the depressing consequences of this difference but, instead, consider for a moment how it actually came about.

ORIGIN OF PRESENT ATTITUDE OF MEDICINE TOWARD MIND

We will not find the origin of the present attitude of medicine toward mind in the earlier chapters of medical history. Ancient physicians would be amazed to learn that, in this golden age of science, what Dr. Adolf Meyer has aptly called a "deadly parallelism" between mind and body could practically exclude mental disorders—major and minor—

from general medical interest. Even our pre-decessors of sixty or seventy years ago knew no such cleavage. Mental diseases were very often the subject of discussion at medical meetings and the mental phenomena observed in general illness were commented upon in as matter-of-fact a way as any others. The interest and determined activity of the New York State Medical Society was responsible for the first state hospital for the insane, the first colony for chronic mental patients and the first institution for the feebleminded in this state. In Connecticut, the first institution for the insane was actually started with a substantial contribution from the State Medical Society, for which the members taxed themselves out of their hard-earned and meagre incomes. The parting of the ways, strange as it may seem, was coincident with the birth of modern scientific medicine.

When new methods of examining diseased organs first engrossed the attention of practitioners and investigators, these methods were applied just as eagerly to mental disorders as they were in an effort to learn the real nature of nephritis, arterial diseases or the acute infections. Those few mental diseases that depend upon demonstrable changes in brain structure became understandable. The nature of general paresis, one of the most prevalent and formidable of mental diseases, for instance, was clearly seen. But new methods of pathological research and the new instruments of precision that were developed for the study of organs in the living threw no light at all upon the main problems of insanity. The absence of demonstrable organic changes in the psychoneuroses—even the severest types— made these disorders seem more mysterious than ever.

The division of man into his organs for the new kind of study made possible by histopathology rendered it more difficult, rather than easier, to understand reactions that involved his total personality. Without such a concept the part played by mind must remain in the realm of metaphysics. The development of hospitals was naturally in the direction of general medical interests and so, to the bitter disappointment of those working in the field of mental diseases, the renaissance of medicine, glorious as it was and much as it meant to suffering humanity, ushered in a period of isolation and neglect for the insane and their problems that is ending only in our own time.

Waning Interest in Function

These are some of the reasons why the rise of scientific medicine was coincident with the establishment of a parallelism that is responsible for the present attitude of medicine toward mind. There is another, however, that stands out above all the rest. This is the rapid decline of scientific interest in *function* not related to *structure* in ways capable of being clearly understood and definitely stated. Functions that are so related were studied, when modern medicine dawned, with increasing enthusiasm and immensely impor-

tant new knowledge concerning them com-
menced to accumulate. No more brilliant
chapter exists in medicine than that which
records the work that provided our present
knowledge of the localization of sensory and
motor functions in brain and spinal cord. But
in the study of functions of mind by the same
methods we find no comparable achievement.
The emotions associated with instinctive activities and the different mental functions grouped
under the concept of intelligence remain practically uncharted in the brain. If medicine
had continued to regard function with its
former interest and respect or with a tiny
part of the interest and respect with which
it came to regard organs, no such parallelism
as that which has been described would exist
to-day. It is here that the gulf between
mental medicine and general medicine is widest
and it is in the practical management of functional disorders, as well as in their scientific
interpretation, that the psychiatrist finds himself most widely separated from his colleagues.

A patient comes to us with a morbid fear. That fear, for all practical purposes, is the most important thing in his life. It profoundly affects all his relations—physiological, family and social. It may result in his death —from suicide perhaps—as surely as carcinoma could. Psychiatry regards that fear as a medical fact, although we are utterly unable, in the present state of knowledge, to correlate it with any structural change in any organ or system of organs and cannot explain its existence or its significance in anatomical, physiological or biochemical terms. Another science, however, psychology, or, to be more precise, a branch of psychology—psychopathology—very largely developed by the study by physicians of mental phenomena in abnormal states, throws light upon the origin of that fear and the part that it plays in the patient's life as a whole. It also provides means for its management so that the fear itself or the dangers that accompany it can be effectively and permanently removed. This

3

would seem to be a creditable medical achievement, but, notwithstanding the fact that the
patient came to a physician for aid, scientific
medicine to-day stands coldly aloof from
everything connected with it.

The sciences of anatomy, physiology, pharmacology, biochemistry, pathology and bacteriology offered no practical help in under-
standing the nature of our patient's fear nor in
its management.   Must we say to him, there-
fore, that those sciences are the sacred and
only foundations of medicine and, until they
reveal the truth, there is no truth that physicians can accept?   Of course we could not do
so logically for, in all other matters, medicine,
in the spirit of scientific investigation, goes
as far afield as necessary.   We unceremon-
iously annex any portion of any science that
will provide weapons for our unending battle
with disease.   Must we, whatever the cost
in human suffering, make psychopathology
the exception because of the theoretical parallelism between mind and body that has

grown up like a noxious weed in the science
and art of medicine? Our patient's morbid
fear and its consequences constitute psychobiological reactions. The anatomical and
physiological part of these reactions will some
day be clearly understood and then, doubtless,
a better method of practical management will
be found than that based upon its psychological nature. But, in the meantime, should
we be inhibited from even attempting to
interpret the psychological phenomena connected with our patient's fear or from using
psychological measures in dealing with it,
unless we are willing to see patient, earnest
work regarded as "unscientific" and, in some
intangible way, "non-medical"? If it is unscientific or non-medical to study psychobiological phenomena until they can be described in anatomical, biochemical or physiological terms, the gulf between workers must
continue to exist until anatomy, physiology
and biochemistry have explanations that now
they are unable to supply. And so with treat-

ment. If it is unscientific or non-medical to employ suggestion, mental analysis, education in the psychology of the emotions, or psychiatric social readjustment in treating the failures in dealing with life that are constituted by mental disorders, either the field of mental medicine must be formally abandoned by trained, scientific physicians or the medical profession, with blind dogmatism, continue to insist upon their forcing psychological issues into physiological ones, regardless of the facts. We must in either case be prepared to see the "no-man's land" that we refuse to occupy over-run by those who are neither inspired by the spirit of scientific investigation nor motivated by the purpose of bringing aid to suffering mankind.

SOME NEW TENDENCIES

If I were compelled to conclude my remarks at this point, I am afraid that I should have accomplished very little in the way of renewing our faith in the strength and symmetry of the structure that we are building.

There are, however, some very significant
events transpiring that may within a few
years transform the unsatisfactory relations
that exist between medicine as a whole and
mental medicine. It should be very clearly
stated that what I have called the "attitude
of medicine toward mind" is the *formal* attitude of medicine and that hundreds of individual physicians—some of them great leaders
—do not share it at all. The old, unproduc-
tive controversy over what is "mental" and
what is "physical" in normal or abnormal
functions is ending. No one can read Can-
non's contributions to our knowledge of such
reactions as rage, hunger and pain without
seeing that only an approach broad enough to
permit them to be considered from the psychobiological point of view throws light upon their
nature. The discovery of regulating mechanisms—chiefly in the central nervous system—
that enable whole systems of organs to act
in harmony with other systems shows us that
the minute study of a single organ is inade-

quate to explain even all of its own functions, much less the part it plays in the life of the organism as a whole. Thus the way is rapidly being cleared for the concept of man as an organism acting, even in his most circum-scribed mental or physical activities, *as a whole*. Sir Charles R. Sherrington, a brilliant student of the relations between functions and organs, in his address as President of the British Association last year, put it this way:

"It is as a whole, a single entity, that the animal —or, for that matter, the plant—has finally and essentially to be envisaged."[3]

It was necessary to take man apart to his last organ for the purpose of studying reactions that take place within himself and to take apart these organs, almost literally to their last cell, to understand their functions in health and the modifications of these func-tions that take place in disease. Now, with the broad psychobiological attitude that Sherrington so clearly formulates, the time

[3] Sherrington, Sir Charles R., "Some aspects of animal mecha-nism," *Science*, September, 29, 1922.

has come to study and treat man again as a
whole. Not only as a "single entity," but
as an organism acting in a social environment
of his own creation, activated by instincts and
regulated by reason, is the re-integrated man
that Sherrington presents to us. How barren
is such a concept with those reactions now
known as "mental" left out of consideration!
It is indeed, as Sherrington said, "to the
psychologist that we must turn to learn in
full the contribution made to the integration
of the animal individual by mind."

Other forces than these trends of scientific
thought are building a bridge between medicine as a whole and that branch of it con-
cerned with mind. One is the eagerness with
which those engaged in other kinds of human-
itarian work accept scientific guidance, thus
opening rich opportunities for the social applications of medicine. In the light provided
by a study of human instinctive tendencies
and the modifications in them made necessary
by the requirements of organized society,

methods have been found to regulate types
of conduct for the control of which there
have been heretofore no better resources than
futile attempts at repression by force alone.
The medical aspects of juvenile delinquency,
crime, drug addiction, prostitution and many
other social ills are much more clearly recognized by lay workers than they used to be.
Until scientific medicine is willing, however,
to accept, *as part of its own body of knowledge*,
the facts regarding human behavior that have
been learned in psychiatry, it will be unable
to assume leadership in the social applications
of its own material.

Medical experiences of the war went far
toward breaking down the isolation of mental
medicine. Physicians in psychiatry had the
opportunity of working side by side with those
engaged in general medical and surgical work,
in the divisions at the front and in base
hospitals. The striking problems created by
the war neuroses were studied under these
novel conditions, but the most important in-

fluence exerted by war experience was the demonstration, upon an immense scale, of the results of managing these problems by several entirely different methods. In one army, where the war neuroses were dealt with, until it was too late to change, in accordance with an erroneous *physiological theory* that ignored psychological factors, the practical results seriously threatened man-power and morale. In another army, where methods of treatment and prevention were based upon *psychological facts*, striking success was achieved.

Another influence that is tending strongly toward undermining the absurd parallelism that lies at the bottom of the conventional attitude of medicine to mind is the increasing interest among psychiatrists in all physical factors in the conditions with which they have to deal. A generous part of even the inadequate appropriations that in so many states are the sole means of support of public institutions for mental diseases is now devoted to diagnostic clinics which compare favorably with those established for dealing with general medical problems elsewhere. In the study of mental deficiency, important work is being done to determine the part played by endocrine disorders and, in the study of the psychoneuroses, physical factors, especially the influence of the vegetative nervous system, are receiving more and more thoughtful attention.

CONCLUSION

Evidence that these influences are, in reality, bringing about a new attitude toward mind in medicine is afforded by the following remark made by Dr. Ray Lyman Wilbur in his address last June as President of the American Medical Association. Speaking particularly of the personal relationship between physician and patient, without which his store of medical knowledge cannot be effectively employed, he said:

"The human mind, the human will and human personality will be as important for the medical student of to-day when he comes to full practice as typhoid fever, small-pox and cholera have been for the physicians in the past. Moral and spiritual qualities play as large a part as do the more physical of the biologic processes."[4]

If that view represents not merely the formulation of an ideal but a practical guide for action, what changes may we not witness during the next few years in medical education, medical practice and medical research!

In research, we shall no longer see two men who are studying different phases of essentially the same biologic process separated by an unseen but impassable wall, simply because one is best fitted by training and experience to use the methods of anatomy, physiology or biochemistry and the other those of psychopathology. Side by side these men will work, employing anatomical, physiological or biochemical terms to describe what they learn from the study of *brain processes* and psychological terms to describe what they learn regarding *mind processes*. One will deal chiefly with states of brain, and the other chiefly with states of mind, but each will be familiar with

[4] Wilbur, Ray Lyman, "Human welfare and modern medicine," *Jour. Am. Med. Assoc.*, June 30, 1923.

the other's point of view and know the value of his approach. Then, and then only, will the mysteries of brain and mind and their relations to each other be revealed.

In practice, the isolation of the insane will be regarded as an absurdity of another age, having nothing but prejudice for its foundation. Suitable wards in our general hospitals will be as freely open to the mentally sick who desire to be cured as they are now to the physically sick. When mental phenomena are encountered in the study or treatment of disease, they will be as thoughtfully and frankly regarded as any other phenomena. Fear, anxiety, compulsive ideas, emotional disorders and anomalies of conduct and of feeling will be, *in fact*, and not merely *by implication*, medical problems. They will be studied from whatever angle the most light can be thrown upon them, instead of being forced into traditional categories or ignored if this process requires too much violence for a gentle art. The charlatan, with his glib use of psychological terms the real meaning of which he is entirely unaware, will be met by science in a field that he now claims for his very own.

In medical education, if, as Dr. Wilbur predicts, "the human mind, the human will and human personality will be as important for the medical student as typhoid fever, small-pox and cholera," a few didactic lectures on insanity will not provide the equipment required. Upon a foundation of knowledge of the mechanisms of mind and their relations, as far as known, with the brain and other organs, will be built an adequate clinical training. The study of mental illness will not have for its clinical material only the most bizarre kinds of situations, studied in strange, non-medical environments. Ordinary people (like ourselves) with ordinary mental problems (like our own) will be studied in ordinary environments so that both student and patient will feel as comfortable in considering those matters that lie at the center of life as they do now in discussing the activities of organs.

In that new kind of medical education that will train physicians to deal with the *total reactions* of human beings—mental and physical and social—I believe that this college is destined to play no unimportant part. The President of the University, the Dean of the College of Physicians and Surgeons and their associates so look upon the function of the modern medical school and soon the material facilities will exist to make their dreams come true. It is certain that when the new school and hospital are opened there will be provisions for the reception and emergency treatment of the mentally ill and for the study—in general wards and clinic—of those mental reactions in common medical and surgical affections that are now, for the most part, passed over merely because they seem to lie outside the formal boundaries of medicine. When that time comes, the physician who graduates from this college will be endowed by his teachers with new and powerful resources not only for the treatment of disease but for its scientific study. The contribution that he can make to social medicine will be vastly increased in effectiveness. Not the least important of the benefits that he will receive, however, may be the ability to see more clearly his own emotional relations to his art and those that determine the attitude of his profession toward its problems.

Bei Fragen zur Produktsicherheit wenden Sie sich bitte an:
If you have any questions regarding product safety,
please contact:

Walter de Gruyter GmbH
Genthiner Straße 13
10785 Berlin
productsafety@degruyterbrill.com